Throat Cancer

Contents

Introduction

Cancer is defined as a disease in which some abnormal body cells multiply and divide without control. As they grow, these cells form different structures, known as tumors.

The throat cancer is a particular type of cancer that appears in the voice box, or it affects the vocal cords, or any other parts of the throat (for example the tonsils or the oropharynx).
There are two main categories of throat cancer: pharyngeal or laryngeal cancer. It can also develop in tonsils.
Pharyngeal cancer, as its name says, develops in the pharynx. The pharynx is that part of the throat that goes from the noes to the top of the windpipe (trachea), in the form of a hollow tube (in the throat). The larynx is also known as the voice box, located just at the top of the trachea/windpipe.

Compared to other types of cancer, throat cancer is relatively uncommon. In USA, approximately 1.1% of the adults are diagnosed with pharyngeal cancer, and around 0.4% of men and women are diagnosed with laryngeal cancer.

Biologically, the throat is a muscular tube, beginning just behind the nose and ending in the neck. Most commonly, throat cancer affects the flat cells that protect the inside of the throat.

The voice box is located just below the throat and can also be affected by throat cancer. It is made out of cartilage and it holds the vocal cords, that vibrate when the persons speaks.
In some cases, throat cancer appears in the piece of cartilage known as epiglottis, the part that is like a lid for the trachea. Also, a form of throat cancer is the one that damages the tonsils, located just on the back of the throat.

Most commonly, cancer of the larynx appears in people aged over 55 years. Also, it occurs among smokers and the most known symptom is hoarseness. It is normally diagnosed with the help of a viewing tube, known as laryngoscope. Its treatment depends on the location and the size of the tumor, but also on the age and the health of the patient. Its treatment includes radiation therapy, surgery or chemotherapy.

It is good to know that in some patients throat cancer includes both pharynx and larynx abnormal growths. In some cases, health professionals consider esophageal cancer a type of throat cancer. In this later situation, the symptoms include pain in the throat and/or in the chest. The illness in this case can be extended from pharynx, to the esophagus, up to the stomach.

Throat cancer symptoms

It is important that any symptoms appear, to see a specialist and try to get a medical opinion on the issue.

In the cases of throat cancer, the most common symptoms include:

➢ Unusual breathing sounds
➢ Cough
➢ Coughing up blood
➢ Difficulty in swallowing
➢ A sensation of hoarseness that does not improve in one or two weeks
➢ Pain in the neck or in the ears
➢ Sore throat that last up to two weeks, even if the patient takes antibiotics
➢ Swelling in the neck
➢ Losing weight without diet

It is not always very easy to detect throat cancer in its early stages. Sometimes, the symptoms include other signs such as:
➤ A different voice
➤ Problems when swallowing (also called dysphagia)
➤ A permanent need to clear the throat
➤ Consistent and persistent cough
➤ Rough breathing

In some cases these symptoms might suggest some other illnesses. But if these signs persist for more than two weeks, a doctor should be seen. Flu symptoms resemble throat cancer symptoms. The most common signs that are similar include:

➤ Cough
➤ Changes in the voice/hoarseness
➤ Pain in the ear
➤ Sore throat.
    However, there is a major difference between flu and throat cancer, as the symptoms in the last case do not go away. Also, the symptoms worsen after two weeks, most likely.

Another classification of throat cancer depends on its location. In this case it can be a cancer in:
1. Nasopharynx: it is in the upper part of the throat, which begins right behind the nose and goes down the neck, up to the esophagus.
2. Oropharynx: it is in the middle part of the throat. It includes the base of the tongue, the soft palate of the back of the mouth, and the tonsils.
3. Hypopharynx: it is in the lower part of the throat, leading to the esophagus. It is the part of the throat that goes to the stomach and the trachea, the tube leading to the lungs.

4. Glottic cancer, affecting the vocal cord.
5. Supraglottic cancer affects the upper part of the larynx, and also affects the epiglottis (a portion of cartilage that prevents food from entering the windpipe)
6. Subglottic cancer develops in the lower part of the voice box, just below the vocal cords.

Cancer developing around the vocal cords (glottis) usually has as symptoms hoarseness or changes in the voice. This helps in an early diagnosis. The recommendation is that if a person has voice changes that do not improve in two weeks, they should see a doctor.

The throat cancer that does not start on the vocal cords, the voice changes appear only at a later stage of the cancer development. These types of cancers are found only when they have already spread to the lymph nodes and the person observes a growing mass in the neck.

The cancers that appear in the area of the larynx, just above the vocal cords (supraglottis) or in the area below the vocal cords (subglottis) do not usually determine voice changes and usually are found in later stages. Their most common symptoms include a sore throat that does not improve, constant coughing, trouble in breathing and in swallowing, ear pain, weight loss and a lump or mass in the neck (because the extension of the cancer near the lymph nodes).

Depending on the particular type of cancer, specific symptoms develop. For example, in the case of mouth cancer, the signs are:
➢ Pain or bleeding in the mouth, that cannot be explained
➢ Pain or swelling in the jaw that does not passes
➢ A sore or an ulcer in the mouth

➤ A sensation of something that is caught in the throat and does not go away

More, any signs of white patches (leukoplakia) or red patches (erythroplakia) in the mouth might suggest pre-malignant cell that can transform into tumors, if they are left untreated.

As said above, some practitioners consider esophageal cancer a type of throat cancer. In this situation, the symptoms are:
➤ Heartburn
➤ The inability to swallow solid food and later, liquid food
➤ The sensation that the food remains in esophagus
➤ Undigested food might be regurgitated
➤ Vomiting blood.

The signs of neck cancer, as a particular form of throat cancer, include:
➤ Loose teeth
➤ A bad breath
➤ Difficulties in hearing
➤ Bleeding in the mouth or throat
➤ The sensation of numbness in the mouth or the lips
➤ A bleeding or persistent blocked nose
➤ Difficulties in breathing or a noisy breathing
➤ White or red patches in the lining of the mouth or the tongue that is not necessarily painful
➤ A loose sense of smell.

These symptoms might lead to an early discovery of throat cancer. However, because they are similar to symptoms of more common illnesses, many of the cancers are discovered in a more advanced stadium.
The symptoms of a more advanced throat cancer are more specific, as it follows:

- The lymph glands in the neck swell, painless at the beginning
- Red or white patches appear in the mouth (on the gums, tongue or the lining of the mouth). Also, the patient might have a swell in the jaw, combined sometimes with unusual bleeding and/or pain.

- The sinuses and the nose can become blocked, and antibiotics have no effect. More, the person has headaches, swollen eyes, pain in the upper teeth and sometimes a bleeding nose.

- An unusual pain in the ear, combined with ringing in the ears and problems in hearing, or even deafness. If the pain in the ear is constant, with a normal swallowing, there is a sign of an infection or a tumor in the throat, most likely.

- Hoarseness in the voice box (larynx), a change in the voice, together with pain felt while swallowing or in the ear. In a more advanced case of cancer, the person has problems in swallowing solid food and cannot breathe easily.

- Swelling around the jawbone or chin, numbness of face muscles, consistent pain in the neck, face and chin.

- In some cases, a symptom is manifested through changes on the skin around the neck area.

More generally, the potential patient should pay a lot of attention to symptoms resembling with the ones described above. It is difficult to diagnose throat cancer in its early stages, also because the symptoms and the signs are different from person to person. Sometimes it is confused with a normal cough or flu and is not very specific.

The symptoms do not stand for a diagnosis, especially in the case of throat cancer. Many other health problems might resemble throat cancer, and any persons developing these signs should discuss their health issues with a health practitioner.

The diagnosis of throat cancer depends on several aspects. First of all, it is analyzed the person's individual history, to find if there are any potential risk factors. Additional test are required, to confirm or exclude the diagnosis of throat cancer.

A list of imaging tests includes CT, MRI, PET scan, X-rays, and barium swallows, but the most useful tool for a definitive diagnosis is a biopsy of the tumor. The biopsy can be done by a surgical incision in the neck, with the help of a fine needle aspiration of the tumor, or by an endoscopic biopsy.

The recommendation is to see a doctor anytime a new symptom appears, or if an older symptom is more persistent. This is important mainly because most of the throat cancer symptoms are not specific to cancer.

Some risks factors are more likely to lead to throat cancer development, especially a given lifestyle habit. The most common are smoking, excessive consumption of alcohol, a deficiency of vitamin A, high exposure to asbestos, or a poor dental hygiene. It was proven that a diet with little fruits and vegetables can also represent a risk for throat cancer, as well as a gastroesophageal reflux disease (GERD).

Research has also shown that throat cancer is most likely to develop at men than at women. More, it was discovered a certain connection between throat cancer and some type of human papillomavirus infections (HPV), a sexually transmitted virus. Cancer Treatment Centers of America acknowledged that HPV infections represent a risk factor for cervical cancers in women and throat cancer.

Moreover, throat cancer can develop in connection with other types of cancers. For example, people diagnosed with throat cancer are also diagnosed with esophageal, lung or bladder cancer in the same time. The reason is that they all have the same risk factors, or in some cases, the cancer starts in one part of the body and extends to other parts of the body.

Another risk factor of throat cancer is smoking and the use of tobacco (including chewing tobacco), associated in many cases with consumption of alcohol, over a long period of time. The combination of smoking and use of alcohol increases the risk of throat cancer. Statistics show that throat cancers are more likely to appear in adults older than 50 years, and 10 times more at men.

The development of throat cancer appears at the point where the cells in that body part suffer genetic mutations. At this point, the cells grow without control and develop into tumors in the throat.

The diagnosis of throat cancer is primarily based on the personal medical history and on the symptoms. However, to confirm the diagnosis, the health professional will perform a laryngoscopy or refer the patient to a specialist especially trained for this type of procedures.

This procedures follows the next steps:

➤ The patient is given a local anesthetic
➤ The doctor inserts a long flexible tube down the throat
➤ With the use of a light and the mirror, the doctors examines the throat
➤ In the case when the test shows abnormalities, the doctor might take a tissue sample from the throat (biopsy) and tests the tissue for cancer.

Throat cancer treatment

As in any treatment for cancer, there are several options, depending on the stage when the cancer is diagnosed, and on some other factors as well.

One option for treatment is surgery. If the tumor found in the throat is small, the doctor might choose to remove it surgically. The operation happens within a hospital and the patient is under sedation.

There are several types of surgeries, depending on the location of the tumor or the stage of the cancer.

➤ Surgery for throat cancer discovered in its early stage. If the tumor is located on the surface of the throat or the vocal cords, it can be removed surgically, with the help of endoscopy. The doctor introduces a hollow endoscope in the patient's throat or in the voice box, and then passes a special surgical tool or a laser through the scope. With the help of these tools, the doctor scrapes off, cut out or vaporize the very superficial cancers.

➤ Surgery made with the purpose to take out all or part of the voice box (laryngectomy). In the case of small tumors, the doctors takes out the part of the voice box that is affected by cancer, leaving as much as possible of the voice box.

Therefore, the doctor aims to preserve the patient's ability to speak and breathe normally. When there is a more-extensive tumor, it might be the case of a total removal of the voice box. The windpipe is then attached to a hole (also called stoma) in the throat to allow the person to breathe (tracheotomy). If the whole larynx is removed, there are several options to restore the ability to speak. The patient should work with a speech pathologist to learn how to speak without a voice box.

➤ Surgery to take out part of the throat (pharyngectomy). It is the situation of small tumors that might require removal of parts of the throat, with the help of surgery. The removed parts can be reconstructed, to allow the patient to swallow food normally afterwards. The surgery to remove large portions of the throat normally includes the removal of the voice box as well.

➤ Surgery to remove lymph nodes that are cancerous (neck dissection). In this situation the throat cancer most likely has spread deeper within the neck, and the doctor would recommend surgery to take out some or all of the lymph nodes, to check if they have cancer cells.

All the surgeries can be minimally invasive, or endoscopic, robotic or with the purpose to remove the tumor and allow the patient a normal functioning in swallowing and speech.

In the cases of any surgical intervention, there are risks of bleeding and infection. Other possible complications are: difficulty speaking or swallowing.

Another possible treatment is radiation therapy. It is normally recommended after surgery. This kind of treatment uses high-energy rays to annihilate malignant cancer cell. Its purpose is to target any cancerous cells left behind after the removal of the tumor, by surgery.

This type of therapy can be external or internal. In the first case, a large machine outside the body (external beam radiation) sends high energy rays, destroying the cancerous cell. In the second case, the radiation is done with the help of small radioactive seeds and wires, placed inside the patient's body, near the cancer (brachytherapy).

Other types are 3D radiation beam therapy and intensity-modulated radiotherapy, tailored to the particular shape of the tumor. The proton therapy is made with the use of a pencil beam technology, pointed directly at the tumor and keeping the nearby tissue healthy.

In the cases when the throat cancer is detected in its early stages, radiation therapy might be the only treatment recommended. In the situations of more advanced throat cancer, radiation therapy is combined with chemotherapy and/or surgery. Also, in these cases radiation therapy reduces the signs and the symptoms and makes the patient more comfortable.

Radiation therapy aimed at the neck may cause side effects:
➢ Sore throat and difficulty swallowing
➢ Changes in the voice

➤ Skin changes in the neck area. These skin changes usually go away when treatment ends.
➤ Changes in the thyroid: Radiation therapy can harm the thyroid (an organ in the neck beneath the voice box). If the thyroid does not make enough thyroid hormone, the patient may feel tired, gain weight, feel cold, and have dry skin and hair. The doctor can check the level of thyroid hormone with a blood test. If the level is low, the patient may need to take thyroid hormone pills
➤ Fatigue. Resting is important, but doctors usually advise people to stay as active as they can.
➤ Weight loss. Some people may need a temporary feeding tube.

A third treatment option is chemotherapy, a type of treatment recommended in the situation when large tumors have extended to the lymph nodes and to other organs or tissue. Chemotherapy is in fact a drug that annihilates and slows down the growth of malignant/cancerous cells.

Some chemotherapy drugs make the patient more sensitive to radiation therapy. The combination of radiation therapy and chemotherapy increases the side effects of both treatments. It is important for the patient to discuss with the doctor about the side effects that the patient is more likely to experience and check if the combined treatments will increase the chances of survival or it will rather worsen the health condition of the person diagnosed with throat cancer.

A fourth type of treatment for throat cancer is the targeted drugs therapy, which takes advantage of given defects of the cancer cells fueling the cells' growth.

One example is Cetuximab (Erbitux), a kind of targeted therapy that has been approved for throat cancer treatment, in some situation. This drug stops the action of the protein which is present in many types of healthy cells, but it is more common in some types of throat cancer cells. Targeted therapy may also interfere with other receptors on cancer cells.

Other targeted drugs are still being under study in clinical trials. Targeted drugs can also be combined with chemotherapy or radiation therapy. In cancer clinical trials, specialists use experimental drugs or other experimental methods that might prove to be successful in reducing the clinical symptoms of throat cancer.

All the treatments referred to above have deep side effects. Therefore, patients should be included in rehabilitation programs after any kind of treatment, working with specialists. The persons that have been under any of this treatment usually face difficulties in swallowing, eating solid foods and talking. The most common issues after throat cancer treatment are:

> Taking care of the surgical opening in the throat (stoma), if the patient had a tracheotomy
> Problems in eating
> Problems in swallowing
> Stiffness and pain in the neck
> Speaking issues.

All the side effects, complication of the treatments and the follow-up scheme, have to be thoroughly discussed with the health care provider.

The treatment of throat cancer is normally approach by a team of doctors, including oncologists, surgeons, plastic surgeons, radiation oncologists, swallowing experts, dentists, speech pathologists, dietitians, therapists (physical, occupational, and speech).

The higher the number of specialists involved in the treatment, the higher is the chance of the patient to be treated accurately and to have increased chances of survival. Moreover, the specialists can find local support groups that would help the patient and the family members to cope with the lifestyle changes required to live well with this kind of illness.

The treatment plan for any patient is customized upon the extent and the seriousness of the throat cancer. Also, it considers bringing to the patient the best chances for a successful outcome.

The treatment should consider preserving the patients' abilities to eat, speak and live a normal life, as much as possible. The treatment plans for throat cancer include one or more of the following approaches: surgery, radiation therapy, chemotherapy, targeted drugs therapies, or a possible participation in the throat cancer clinical trials.

The treatment of throat cancer includes in most of the case some lifestyle changes and use of home remedies. If the patient is smoking for example, one of the acknowledged causes of throat cancer, the patient has to quit. Giving up smoking presents a series of benefits:

➢ It increases the effectiveness of treatment
➢ Makes it easier for the body to heal after surgery

➢ Decreases the chances of getting another cancer in the future.

For many people, quitting smoking is rather difficult, especially in such a stressful situation as it is cancer diagnosis. However, the patient can discuss their options with health professionals, and can use medication, nicotine replacement products and/or go to counseling.

The other high risk factor, which is consumption of alcohol, should also be eliminated. When the patient stops drinking alcohol, it decreases the risks of a second cancer and allows the body to better tolerate the cancer treatments.

Even if there is no certainty that other alternative treatments might work in the cure of throat cancer, any patient can seek help in complementary and alternative cures. Most likely they will help the patient deal with side effects of the classical throat cancer treatment.

The most common options of alternative treatment include:
➢ Acupuncture
➢ Massage therapy
➢ Meditation
➢ Relaxation techniques

Throat cancer survival

A very important aspect of the throat cancer survival is the coping and the support part. The cancer diagnosis is a difficult issue for every person, because it affects a part of the body extremely important for everyday activities (breathing, eating, and talking). Moreover, the patients tend to become even more worried about the side effects of the treatment plans and the chances for survival.

Most of the persons diagnosed with throat cancer have the feeling that the situation is out of their hands. To deal with this situation, patients are advised to consider the following:

➢ To find out as much as they can about throat cancer, so they can take the most suitable decisions in terms of treatment. Any questions might appear should be discussed with the doctor. Also, the patient is advised to ask about further sources of information about cancer. When the person knows more about their condition, they are more comfortable when making treatment decisions.

➢ To speak with someone else about throat cancer. The sources of support are extremely important in helping the patient deal with the emotions they are feeling. In some cases patients choose to speak with a close friend or a family member that is a very good listener. In some other situations, patients seek out for help at clergy members or counselors.

➢ It is important for the patient to take care of themselves during the cancer treatment. It is a priority to keep the body healthy during the treatment and to avoid additional stress. It is recommended for the patient to get enough sleep each night, to keep feeling rested. Also, sometimes they can take a walk or exercise, if they feel comfortable with it. Relaxing, listening to music or reading a book is suitable and easy way to keep a good mood.

➢ The person diagnosed with throat cancer should go to all the follow-up meetings. The doctor will appoint follow-up examinations every few months for the first two years after treatment and with lower frequency afterwards. During these examinations, the doctors monitors the recovery of the patient and checks for a cancer recurrence.

Even if the follow-up exams could make the patient nervous, as they remind of the hard period of treatment, anxiety will go away in time. It is recommended to plan in advance relaxing activities to help redirect the fears of the patient.

For patients that have survived cancer, different methods of support are available. First of all, they receive rehabilitation support in terms of physical, occupational, and speech therapy. Other persons may need additional surgical treatment, as it is for example reconstructive surgery and/or dental implants.

Also, speech pathologists, audiologists, and experts in swallowing rehabilitation might be needed. Support groups are extremely helpful altogether.

There are different prognoses for persons diagnosed with throat cancer and they depend on the stage and the location of the cancer. Most of the survival indicators rely on a 5-year relative survival rate, which vary with the type of cancer and its stage.

The higher survival rates were registered in the case of the glottis cancer (90%), and the worst survival rate is in the case of hypopharynx cancer (53%), both of them beginning at stage 1 over a 5-year period. In all individuals diagnosed with throat cancer, the 5-year survival rates decreases, as the stages progress from 1 to 4. However, the earlier the cancer is diagnosed and treated, the higher is the survival rate.

In terms of prevention, there is no available cancer screening at this moment. It is recommended that those persons that present higher risk for throat cancer to see a doctor if any symptoms persist. Also, the persons with increased risks, or the ones who smoke, or have been exposed to HPV, asbestos, nickel, or sulfuric acid fumes, should check their health status, for an early discovery of throat cancer.

The avoidance of risky situation also decreases the chances of getting throat cancer, but there is no guarantee that it can fully be prevented. Nevertheless, the vaccine against HPV in young men and women reduces the cancer risk.

In terms of survival rates, there are available data for laryngeal and hypopharyngeal cancer, by stages. It is calculated in terms of the percentage of patients who live at least 5 years after the cancer is diagnosed.

The 5 year relative survival rates compare the survival rates for the people with cancer to the rates for people without it. It is important to know that many of the patients live much longer than 5 years after their cancer is found and treated. The rates are calculated based on the stage of the cancer at its discovery moment.

The numbers are offered by the National Cancer Data Base, from United States of America, based on patients diagnosed between 1998-1999, and were published in 2010. They offer an overall picture, but they should be analyzed with attention, because some treatments have improved since then, and of course, the survival rate depends from person to person.

Survival rates in case of **supraglottis cancer** (the larynx above the vocal cords, including the epiglottis):

Stage	5-year relative survival rates
I	59%
II	59%
III	53%
IV	34%

Survival rates for **glottis cancer** (the part of the larynx that includes the vocal cords)

Stage	5-year relative survival rates
I	90%
II	74%
III	56%
IV	44%

Survival rates for **subglottis cancer** (the larynx below the vocal cords)

Stage	5-year relative survival rates
I	65%
II	56%
III	47%
IV	32%

Survival rates for **hypopharynx** (the area around the vocal cords)

Stage	5-year relative survival rates
I	53%
II	39%
III	36%
IV	24%

Throat cancer stages

Depending on the how developed are the cancerous cells in the patient's body, there are several stages of the throat cancer. Each of it refers to the extent of the cancer.

There are several stages, as it follows:
  - ➤ **Stage 0:** the tumor is small and has not extended yet to the throat;
  - ➤ **Stage 1:** the tumor is under 7 cm and is located only in the throat;

> **Stage 2:** the tumor is very little larger than 7 cm, and remains limited to the throat;
> **Stage 3:** the tumor is bigger and extended beyond the throat tissue, to other organs;
> **Stage 4:** the tumor has spread to the lymph nodes and/or other distant organs.

The stage of the cancer is established with the help of imaging test like a CT scan or an MRI. These show a good picture of the progression of the cancer, the doctor looking at the chest, neck and head of the patient.

To identify the stage of the throat cancer, the health professional makes use of the following methods:

> Endoscopy, with a special lighted scope. At the end of the endoscope is a small camera which transmits images of the throat to a video screen, where the doctor looks for signs of abnormalities. Another type of scope (laryngoscope) can be inserted in the patient's voice box. It uses magnifying lens, through which the doctor examines the vocal cords.

> Testing of a tissue sample for abnormalities. The sample is taken during an endoscopy or a laryngoscopy, in which the doctor passes surgical instruments through the scope, to collect the tissue. The sample is tested in laboratory, for cancer.

> The extent of the cancer can be identified with the help of imaging tests, such as X-ray, computerized tomography (CT), magnetic resonance imaging (MRI), and positron emission tomography (PET).

The stage of the cancer is the most relevant factor in deciding upon the treatment option. Every treatment plan is realized individually. Also, if the cancer was discovered at an early point, the doctors review the pathology, to check if the diagnosis and the stage were correctly confirmed. If the cancer is in fact a recurrence, more comprehensive testing is made, to make an adapted treatment plan.

Throat cancer pain

Nevertheless, throat cancer causes pain and determines important life changes. However, there are several approaches that manage cancer pain, depending on its severity. The World Health Organization developed a 3-step plan for cancer pain management, with the use of medication:

1. For mild and moderate pain, the patient could take a nonsteroidal anti-inflammatory drug (NSADs). Patients must be monitored with attention for side effects, such as problems in kidney, heart, and blood vessel, or stomach and intestinal problems.

2. If the pain increases in intensity and duration, the prescription for pain killers is chanced. For every step, the doctors prescribe regular doses, which are taken on given times. This way, the patient is prevented from becoming addicted, and a controllable dose of medication is kept in the patient's body.

In these cases, the medication is given in oral administration, or by infusion or injection. In some situations, if the pain appears between the scheduled doses of drug, the doctor might prescribe additional doses.

The medication for pain is prescribed individually for each patient's circumstances and physical condition. For the relief of moderate to severe pain, NSAIDs might be prescribed together with opioids. Especially older patients should be closely monitored if they are under such medication plan. It is not recommended to give aspirin to children, to treat pain.

3. Opioids are extremely effective in treating moderate and severe pain. However, on a long term basis, patients with cancer tend to become tolerant to them. In such moments, the doctor increases the doses. It should not be confused the opioid or physical dependence on it with addiction (which is the psychological dependence).

Here are some examples of opioids: morphine (the most commonly used in cancer pain treatment), hydromorphone, oxycodone, methadone, fentanyl, and tramadol.

Opioids are taken only on a regular fixed schedule, and only when the pain appears outside the schedule, the dose is increased. The dose depends on the chosen opioid. The proper dosage of opioid is established to the next principle: it is given the lowest dose that controls pain, with the fewest side effects. The purpose is to reach to a balance between the pain relief and the side effects, with a gradual adjustment of the dose.

The pain medication can be administered in several manners: by mouth, if the patient has no stomach problems, rectally, through medication patches placed on the skin. Other methods are intravenous, or the medication is given through the Patient-controlled analgesia (PCA) pumps. In the situation when the patients have uncontrollable pain, opioids are given intraspinal, in combination with a local anesthetic.

The regular use of opioids may cause one or all of the following side effects:

➢ Nausea
➢ Sleepiness
➢ Constipation
➢ Vomiting
➢ Difficulty in thinking clearly
➢ Problems in breathing

The pain medication can also be administered in combination with some other drugs, such as antidepressants, anticonvulsants, local anesthetics, corticosteroids, bisphosphonates, and stimulants.

To keep in mind: the medication plan is attentively and closely discussed with the doctor, and any side effect should be reported immediately.

The cancer pain can be treated with the help of some other physical and psychosocial interventions. These can be used together with medication or any other treatment of pain management. Nevertheless, every patient is treated individually and has their personal treatment plan.

Physical interventions include:

> Heat (a heating pad) for weakness, muscle wasting, muscle/bone pane
> Cold (flexible ice packs)
> Massage
> Pressure
> Vibration, for an increased relaxation
> Exercising for strengthening the weak muscles, loosen joint, strengthening of the heart and restoration of the coordination and balance
> Changes in the patient's position
> Restriction of movement of areas that are painful

Other types of interventions for treating cancer pain address the thinking and the behavior of the patients. These treatments give patients the sense of control and enhance in them the coping skills to deal with the cancer and its signs.

The thinking and behavioral interventions which begin in the early stage of the diagnosis help the patients to learn and practice the skills, when they have enough strength and energy.

The thinking and behavioral interventions include:
> Relaxation and imagery

> Hypnosis (these techniques helps the patients relax and can be combined with other methods). It is efficient in easing the pain especially in patients that are able to focus and use imagery, and, of course, are willing to use this technique

➢ Redirecting thinking: the attention is focused on some other triggers than pain or other feelings that come with it. The distractions can be internal (praying, for example), or external (such as listening to music, watching television, talking, listening to someone that reads to them). Also, patients can be taught to evaluate their negative thoughts and to replace them with more positive images.

➢ Patient education. In this case, the health care providers give instructions and lots of information about the cancer, to both the patients and the patients' families. Barriers that stop effective pain management are also discussed.

➢ Psychological support, such as short-term psychological therapy, to prevent clinical depression or any adjustment disorder.

➢ Support groups and religious counseling.

In treating the cancer pain, doctors might proceed to some more invasive interventions, especially when less invasive methods have no effective results.

The invasive interventions are:

➢ Nerve blocking, with the help of an injection of a local anesthetic or a drug that inactivates nerves that control the pain.

➢ Neurologic interventions, with the help of surgery. The intervention implies the implantation of devices that deliver drugs in the body, or electrically stimulate the nerves. In extreme cases, surgery is used to annihilate nerves that are causing the pain.

In the cancer treatment, the pain is also caused by the treatment procedures, and not by the cancer itself. In these situations, the doctors use anesthetics or short-acting opioids, together with anti-anxiety drugs and sedatives.

It is known that patients tolerate the pain throughout medical procedures if they are explained what to expect. More, some patients prefer to have a relative or a friend staying with them during the procedure, to help reduce the anxiety.

It is part of the cancer pain management to inform the patient and the family members as well, how to treat pain at home.

Suggestions of relaxations exercises, to relieve cancer pain:

Exercise 1: slow rhythmic breathing

- Breathe in slowly and deeply, keeping the stomach and shoulders relaxed.
- As the person breathes out slowly, they begin to relax, as the tension leaves the body
- Breathe in and out slowly and regularly at a comfortable rate. Let the breath come all the way down to the stomach, as it completely relaxes.
- To help the focus on the breathing and to breathe slowly and rhythmically: Breathe in as you say silently to yourself, "in, two, three." OR Each time you breathe out, say silently to yourself a word such as "peace" or "relax."

➢ Do steps 1 through 4 only once or repeat steps 3 and 4 for up to 20 minutes.
➢ End with a slow deep breath.

Exercise 2: simple touch, massage, or warmth for relaxation:
➢ Brief touch or massage, such as hand holding or briefly touching or rubbing a person's shoulders

➢ Soaking feet in a basin of warm water or wrapping the feet in a warm, wet towel

➢ Massage (3 to 10 minutes) of the whole body or just the back, feet, or hands. If the patient is modest or cannot move or turn easily in bed, consider massage of the hands and feet

➢ Use a warm lubricant. A small bowl of hand lotion may be warmed in the microwave oven or a bottle of lotion may be warmed in a sink of hot water for about 10 minutes

➢ Massage for relaxation is usually done with smooth, long, slow strokes

➢ Especially for the elderly person, a back rub that effectively produces relaxation may consist of no more than 3 minutes of slow, rhythmic stroking (about 60 strokes per minute) on both sides of the spine, from the crown of the head to the lower back. Continuous hand contact is maintained by starting one hand down the back as the other hand stops at the lower back and is raised. Set aside a regular time for the massage. This gives the patient something pleasant to anticipate.

Exercise 3: Peaceful past experiences

The patient could think of the following questions:
- Can you remember any situation, even when you were a child, when you felt calm, peaceful, secure, hopeful, or comfortable?
- Have you ever daydreamed about something peaceful? What were you thinking?
- Do you get a dreamy feeling when you listen to music? Do you have any favorite music?
- Do you have any favorite poetry that you find uplifting or reassuring?
- Have you ever been active religiously? Do you have favorite readings, hymns, or prayers? Even if you haven't heard or thought of them for many years, childhood religious experiences may still be very soothing.

Exercise 4: Active listening to recorded music

- Choose a type of music you like. Most people prefer fast, lively music, but some select relaxing music. Other options are comedy routines, sporting events, old radio shows, or stories
- Keep your eyes open and focus on a fixed spot or object. If you wish to close your eyes, picture something about the music
- Listen to the music at a comfortable volume. If the discomfort increases, try increasing the volume; decrease the volume when the discomfort decreases.
- If this is not effective enough, try adding or changing one or more of the following: massage your body in rhythm to the music; try other music; or mark time to the music in more than one manner, such as tapping your foot and finger at the same time.

Throat cancer statistics

Throat cancer is affecting a great number of people worldwide. Statistics show how many people have been diagnosed with throat cancer, what the average age at diagnosis is, and how many persons are still alive at a given time of the treatment. Also, statistics show the patients profile in terms of age, sex, racial/ethnic group, geographic location, and other factors.

Statistical trends about throat cancer are useful for governments, policy makers, health professionals, and researchers, who seek to understand the impact of cancer on the population and what strategies are more suitable for its treatment and prevention.

Statistics about cancer in United States of America:
➤ It is estimated that in 2016, around 1, 7 million new case of cancer will be diagnosed, and almost 600,000 people will die of it.

➤ The most common cancers are: breast cancer, lung and bronchus cancer, prostate cancer, colon and rectum cancer, bladder cancer, melanoma of the skin, non-Hodgkin lymphoma, thyroid cancer, kidney and renal pelvis cancer, leukemia, endometrial cancer, and pancreatic cancer.

➤ The number of new cases of cancer (cancer incidence) is 454.8 per 100,000 men and women per year (based on 2008-2012 cases)

> The number of cancer deaths (cancer mortality) is 171.2 per 100,000 men and women per year (based on 2008-2012 deaths)

> Cancer mortality is higher among men than women (207.9 per 100,000 men and 145.4 per 100,000 women). It is highest in African American men (261.5 per 100,000) and lowest in Asian/Pacific Islander women (91.2 per 100,000). (Based on 2008-2012 deaths.)

> The number of people living beyond a cancer diagnosis reached nearly 14.5 million in 2014 and is expected to rise to almost 19 million by 2024

> Approximately 39.6 percent of men and women will be diagnosed with cancer at some point during their lifetimes (based on 2010-2012 data)

> In 2014, an estimated 15,780 children and adolescents ages 0 to 19 were diagnosed with cancer and 1,960 died of the disease

> National expenditures for cancer care in the United States totaled nearly $125 billion in 2010 and could reach $156 billion in 2020.

Statistics about cancer worldwide show the following:

> Cancer is among the leading causes of death worldwide. In 2012, there were 14 million new cases and 8.2 million cancer-related deaths worldwide

> The number of new cancer cases will rise to 22 million within the next two decades

➢ More than 60 percent of the world's new cancer cases occur in Africa, Asia, and Central and South America; 70 percent of the world's cancer deaths also occur in these regions.

Specifically in the case of throat/head and neck cancer or oral cancer, the statistics show the following:

➢ Head and neck cancer accounts for about 3% of all cancers in the United States. In 2016, an estimated 61,760 people (45,330 men and 16,430 women) will develop head and neck cancer

➢ It is estimated that 13,190 deaths (9,800 men and 3,390 women) will occur in 2016

➢ Oropharyngeal cancer is the eleventh most common cancer worldwide

➢ Incidence and mortality rates are higher in men than women. Differences across countries particularly relate to distinct risk profiles and availability and accessibility of health services

➢ Tobacco use, including smokeless tobacco, and excessive alcohol consumption are estimated to account for about 90% of oral cancers

The appointment with the doctor

If a person notices any of the symptoms described above, one or more, they should see a doctor to establish what it might be. The doctor that is specialized in diseases and conditions affecting the ears, nose or throat is called otolaryngologist.

The preparation for the appointment with the health provider includes:

> Taking into consideration any pre-appointment restrictions (for example in terms of diet)
> Writing down all the symptoms that the patient has experience, even the ones that seem irrelevant
> Keeping an evidence of key personal information, such as recent life changes
> Keeping an evidence of all the medications or supplements the patient is taking.

During the appointment, the patient should keep in mind to get informed in the following aspects:

> What is likely causing the symptoms or condition?
> Are there other possible causes for the symptoms or condition?
> What kinds of tests do they need?
> What is the best course of action?
> What are alternative treatments?
> Are there any restrictions to follow?

Meanwhile, the doctor most likely will ask the person the following:

➢ When did the person first begin experiencing symptoms?
➢ Have the symptoms been continuous or occasional?
➢ How severe are the symptoms?
➢ What, if anything, seems to improve the symptoms?
➢ What, if anything, appears to worsen the symptoms?

Prevention of throat cancer

Until now, nothing was proven to effectively prevent throat cancer to appear. However, in order to reduce the risks, it is recommended to:

➢ Quitting smoking or not smoking at all
➢ Drinking alcohol in moderation. For women this is one drink a day, for men it means no more than two drinks a day
➢ Following a healthy diet, rich in fruits in vegetables
➢ Protection from HPV (limiting the number of sexual partners, use of condoms, and HPV vaccine, available to boys, girls, and young women and men.

Relevant info about throat cancer

...if the cancer is diagnosed in its early stages, it has a high survival rate

...the throat cancer is not treatable once it has spread to other parts of the body, beyond the neck and the head

...treatment of throat cancer (like in the case of any cancer) prolongs the patient's life and slows down the progression of the cancer

...after treatment, some persons need therapy to learn again how to eat and to speak. The health state improves by working with a speech therapist and a physical therapist.

...some patients might experience complications, such as disfigurement of the neck or the face, inability to speak, difficulty in breathing, or skin hardening around the neck

...alternative names of throat cancer are: Vocal cord cancer; Throat cancer; Laryngeal cancer; Cancer of the glottis; Cancer of oropharynx or hypopharynx

... Cancers arising in the larynx (voice box) are devastating malignancies that account for roughly 200,000 deaths annually worldwide. Although this only represents 2-5% of all malignancies, these cancers have special importance because of their significant effects on voice, swallowing and quality of life

... In the United States, it is estimated that over 12,000 new cases are diagnosed each year and that this incidence is increasing during a time that many other cancers are decreasing

... Tobacco use is known to be the major predisposing factor for laryngeal cancer

...alcohol use, nutritional deficiencies, genetic predisposition and viral factors may also play a role

... The vast majority (85-90%) of cancers of the larynx are squamous cell carcinomas that arise from the covering of the vocal cords

...modern treatment approaches have become more and more complex, and researchers developed sophisticated methods to try to preserve the vocal function of the throat cancer patients

... Early cancer of the glottis (vocal cords) or supraglottis (false vocal cords) can be effectively treated with either surgery alone or radiation therapy

...Most surgical procedures can spare major portions of the voice box and with modern techniques; reconstruction of the voice box can be accomplished with preservation of reasonable voice quality and swallowing

... The past ten years have seen the introduction of laser resections for many of these cancers thereby avoiding external neck incisions

...cancers that are superficial or limited in extent are best treated with laser removal. Similar tumors are also easily cured with 6-7 weeks of radiation treatment

...deeply invasive cancers are best treated with surgical excision, often combined with modified or selective neck dissection (removal of lymph nodes). Most of these procedures can preserve some vocal function without permanent tracheostomy

...Superficial cancers or those of smaller volume can be effectively treated with radiation alone, but local recurrence rates are higher than with primary surgery

...Standard treatment for patients with advanced laryngeal cancer has historically consisted of total laryngectomy, often combined with modified neck dissection

...When metastatic cancer is present in the lymphatics of the neck, surgery is combined with radiation therapy

...Five-year cure rates vary from 40-60%. The major sequelae of total laryngectomy include loss of natural voice and problems associated with living with a permanent tracheal stoma (hole in the neck)

...Modern voice restoration techniques with tracheoesophageal puncture (Blom-Singer prosthesis) has significantly reduced loss of voice as a result of total laryngectomy since the majority of patients are able to speak with a naturally sounding, lung powered voice and fewer patients must rely on the electrolarynx or esophageal speech

...The selection of treatment therefore depends on a balance between side effects, experience of the treating physicians, cost and patient desire

…None of the newer treatment approaches have demonstrated improvements in survival rates compared to total laryngectomy

…between 2003 to 2012, cancer death rates decreased by:
> ➢ 1.8 percent per year among men
> ➢ 1.4 percent per year among women
> ➢ 2.0 percent per year among children ages 0-19

…Although death rates for many individual cancer types have also declined, rates for a few cancers have stabilized or even increased.

…As the overall cancer death rate has declined, the number of cancer survivors has increased. These trends show that progress is being made against the disease, but much work remains.
…Although rates of smoking, a major cause of cancer, have declined, the U.S. population is aging, and cancer rates increase with age. Obesity, another risk factor for cancer, is also increasing

…Benign tumors (such as polyps or nodules): are usually not a threat to life; can be treated or removed and usually don't grow back; do not invade the tissues around them; do not spread to other parts of the body

…Malignant growths: may be a threat to life; usually can be treated or removed but can grow back; can invade and damage nearby tissues and organs; can spread to other parts of the body

…A biopsy is the only sure way to know if the abnormal area is cancer

...CT scan: An x-ray machine linked to a computer takes a series of detailed pictures of your neck, chest, or abdomen. You may receive an injection of contrast material so your lymph nodes show up clearly in the pictures. CT scans of the chest and abdomen can show cancer in the lymph nodes, lungs, or elsewhere.

...MRI: A large machine with a strong magnet linked to a computer is used to make detailed pictures of your neck, chest, or abdomen. MRI can show cancer in the blood vessels, lymph nodes, or other tissues in the abdomen.

Thank You for reading this book. I would be really appreciated if you could rate it on **Amazon.com**. Thanks again!